To HIIT or Not to HIIT

Why You Should Consider HIIT Training

Vincent Blackshear

ISBN: 1548296244
ISBN-13: 978-1548296247

Table of Contents

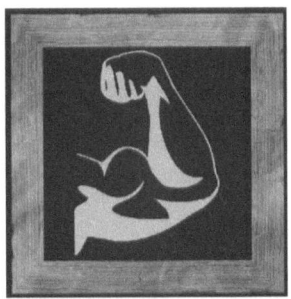

Introduction

You're about to discover the benefits of High Intensity Interval Training or what is popularly known today as HIIT. Imagine reaping the benefits of a full cardio workout but only spending as little as 15 minutes instead of a full hour.

That's only one of the benefits of this mode of training. However, they don't call it "intense" for nothing. It's going to be painful, it's going to make you want to give up, it's the kind of training that goes all or nothing.

This book will go over the pros and cons of HIIT training, why it's so popular, and the factors that you need to consider before you decide whether it's the kind of workout for you or not.

This book will also cover some of the mistakes that people make when they undergo a HIIT session. You will learn why some people end up giving up on HIIT workouts and miss out on the benefits of this training method. We will also dispel the most common myths about HIIT training and give you the plain simple truth.

Thank you and I hope you enjoy it!

VINCENT BLACKSHEAR

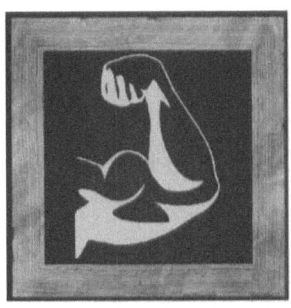

Chapter 1

What is HIIT

HIIT stands for high intensity interval training. It is all a-buzz in the health and fitness world. People just call them HIIT workouts or sprint interval training or high intensity intermittent exercise or some other fancy sounding name.

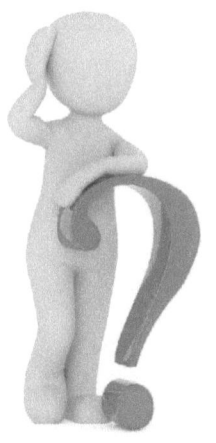

They all mean the same thing. Let's just call them HIIT workouts or HIIT training for short. First off, let's get this part out of the way – this type of training or workout will be somewhat similar or akin to a form of cardio.

Okay, some folks who have been trying to lose weight for quite a while will tell you that cardio really has very minimal effects on weight loss. That's what you will hear from people who have been struggling with weight loss especially those who have done countless hours on a treadmill.

Some would say it doesn't work – well, we'll get to HIIT vs. steady state cardio quite shortly but we have to get one thing out of the way first.

HIIT is totally something else. It's not your run off the mill cardio. Unlike the steady monotonous cardio exercises that people have been doing in the past decade, this one is actually backed by actual science.

HIIT workouts are a time efficient and potent form of interval training that can induce metabolic adaptations in the body. It helps you improve your ability to perform exercises that mainly rely on aerobic energy metabolism.

Your overall performance is improved. However, that is not the only effect. Studies have shown that doing HIIT training regimens can improve your body's peak oxygen uptake. And in the body's skeletal muscles, it increases their maximal activity.

That means an increase in the energy metabolism of your skeletal muscles and your body's overall capacity to keep on exercising. Because your body has the capacity to adapt, it is forced to make them quickly with this type of interval training. You get better results in a shorter period of time.

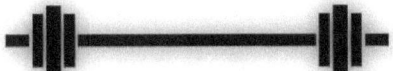

The Training Technique

HIIT is a type of interval training. That means you will be switching from one phase of training to another and then back again. In one phase of training you will be giving your 100% effort (or something as close to that as possible – big grin!) in the given exercise at hand. In this phase you will do exercises in intense bursts of effort – and when we say intense, we mean really intense.

After the 100% effort phase, you will switch to a recovery period. This recovery period is only very short. It is also usually active, which means you will still be exercising but with minimal intensity. It is more of a relaxed phase than a resting phase actually.

After this short recovery phase, you will then switch back to the intense burst phase. You will then switch back and forth between these two phases until your training session is completed.

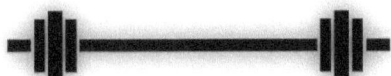

The Effects of HIIT Training

A lot of bodybuilders will recognize this training pattern used in HIIT workouts. Well, partly because if you just tweak or shorten the rest or recovery cycles in bodybuilding you will get an HIIT workout.

You get to burn more body fat using training that is comparably shorter. That means this form of training is definitely more efficient compared to static or steady state exercises. Studies have shown that training in this manner will keep your heart rate up longer.

According to experts like the Fhitting Room's Eric Salvador (NSCA, NASM), this type of high intensity exercise creates an oxygen shortage in the body. This means that during the intense effort, your body will require more oxygen than usual. That's how intense the workouts should be.

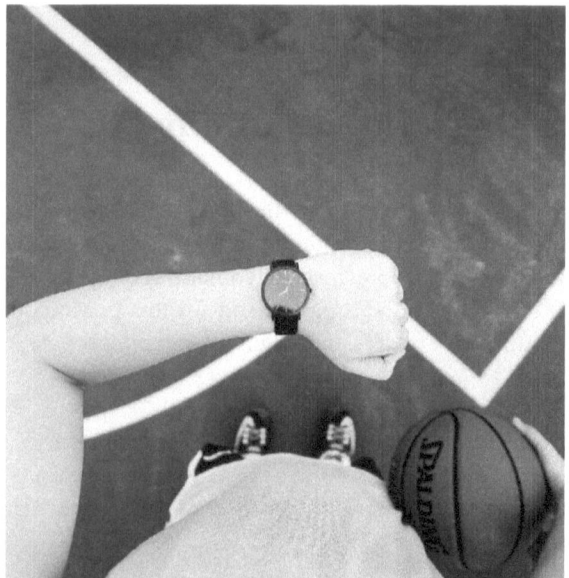

This increased oxygen requirement creates a shortage, which means your body will be asking for more oxygen even after you are done with your workout. It's like getting an after burn even when you're just resting an hour later. You will still be burning calories after putting on your street clothes.

This after burn effect is called Excess Post Exercise Oxygen Consumption or EPOC for short. This EPOC effect is the reason why intense exercises like HIIT training is so much better for weight loss compared to regular steady state exercises and aerobic exercises.

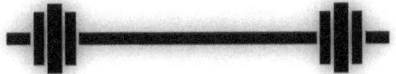

Advantages of HIIT Training

Here are some of the advantages of HIIT workouts compared to aerobic and other cardio exercises.

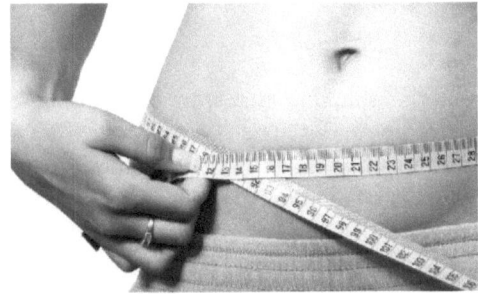

- **Little to No Equipment Needed:** this is one of the best things about high intensity interval training. You don't necessarily need exercise equipment to get it done. A lot of the exercises you will be doing will be comparable to plyometrics (well, some HIIT routines also incorporate plyometrics). You don't have a dumbbell? No problem. You can still do HIIT. You have a few weights around? Sure, you can still use them in HIIT training.

- **Convenient and Time Conscious:** So, you don't have a lot of time to work out – busy schedule, right? Do you have 30 minutes to spare each day? Maybe, 15 minutes? Cutting it close, do you have 10 minutes? Simply put, gone are the days when excuses like "I don't have time" really make sense. You get a maximum calorie burn in just a fraction of the time (yes, it does sound like an infomercial – big grin! But it works!)

- **You Exercise Anywhere:** Going to the gym to get a really good work out can sometimes be can sometimes be an inconvenience. The good news is that you don't need to go to the gym to get your

7

HIIT workout done. Of course, you can go to the gym and do your routine there or you can go to the park, do it in the hotel room where you're staying during your business trip, at home, or in your garage if you have some space there.

- **<u>Increase Your Body's Metabolism:</u>** When you combine interval training with high intensity exercises you achieve the state called EPOC. Your metabolic rate shoots up like crazy. Do you know how long an EPOC state can last? Some HIIT routines are so intense your body will still be burning fat even after 48 hours after your workout.

Now, you may be thinking that you can get these same benefits by simply doing a cardio workout. The short answer to that question is both a yes and a no – yes, it can be that confusing sometimes. If you want to really understand why that is so, you need to get the detailed and long answer. To get the long answer to that lingering question in the minds of other folks, we will go over regular cardio versus HIIT workouts in the next chapter.

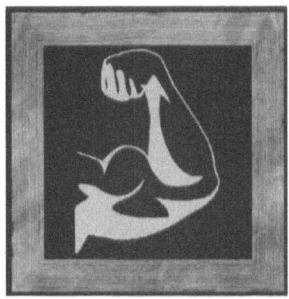

Chapter 2

HIIT versus Cardio

In the previous chapter we have touched on some of basic details about high intensity interval training. As stated earlier, this type of training will make you do repeated bouts or exercises that have a higher intensity than other exercises. After each intense exercise period follows a short period of recovery which is usually active but not as intense. That means your body switches from high intensity to medium or low intensity.

The intense periods range from a few seconds to several minutes. Some intense exercises will only require you to perform a bout or intense feat for about 5 seconds or less. Well, there are exercises that will require an intense performance that will last for 8 minutes or a bit more.

Experts recommend that you should perform these intense exercises at 80% to 95% of your maximal heart rate. That basically refers to the maximum number of times your heart will beat in just one minute without necessarily overexerting yourself.

That means you will have to measure your heart rate when you are resting and while you are exercising. You will also measure your maximum heart rate per minute as well. You'll go over these numbers with your fitness instructor or HIIT trainer.

Note that some recovery periods can be made just as long as the high intensity period. These exercises are more forgiving – however, there are HIIT workouts that are not as gentle (if that is a good word to call it).

The rest periods or periods of low to medium intensity will require you to perform the exercises at 40% or even 50% of your maximal heart rate (it will vary from one HIIT workout routine to another).

As stated in the previous chapter, HIIT routines will vary when it comes to training time. Some will only require less than 10 minutes (especially if the routine is for beginners) while others will require twice as many minutes of working out. There are training routines that can last for 30 minutes to an hour.

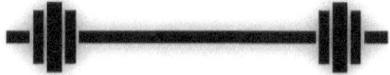

So How Is That Different From Cardio?

Note that when we say "cardio exercises" we are generally referring to steady state cardio exercises. Those are the exercises that elevate your heart rate and the intensity of the exercise usually just remains constant.

Think of your regular jogging in the morning or afternoon, cycling, or perhaps working out on a treadmill. You usually follow the same routine and maintain the same level of intensity all throughout your training regime. Some days you may increase the intensity but it rarely varies.

The result of course is that you burn calories. There is no arguing that. Staying active always pays off compared to being a couch potato and doing nothing. Will steady state cardio help you live longer – of course; absolutely.

What we know so far (and this is general knowledge already by the way) is that any type of moderate physical activity – like a daily thirty minute walk or brisk walking – will greatly improve your longevity compared to living a sedentary lifestyle.

That alone is beneficial even to people who have health risks like diabetes, high blood pressure, or a smoking habit. Incorporating even a simple activity like a regular jog or walk can greatly improve their health condition. The trick is to do it on a regular basis – make it a regular part of your life.

Even people who are on a diet will attest that any exercise program will help them lose weight and stay on the path mandated by their diets. Regular exercise alone (referring to steady state cardio as well) is enough to lower hypertension. It already helps your body to develop denser and stronger bones, improve your body's cholesterol levels, and control blood sugar.

IMPORTANT POINT: We are not ranting against steady state cardio in this book. We aren't even saying that you should ditch your steady state cardio. Don't sign out of your taebo, aerobics, zumba, gym time, or any other workout you may already be involved with.

That's already great. Keep it up. What we are saying is that you can incorporate HIIT into your workout regimen to get better results and make your workout more efficient.

Now, who doesn't want faster results in the shortest time possible?

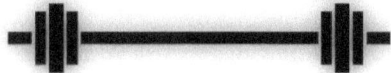

HIIT vs. Steady State Cardio Intensity

They wouldn't call it "high intensity" interval training if it wasn't intense, right? This level of fitness activity can be pretty challenging especially for beginners. Of course, HIIT workouts can be adjusted for people of different fitness levels. However, that doesn't take away the fact that the level of the exercises done in these workouts can be quite difficult for someone who hasn't done any exercising in a while.

Steady state cardio on the other hand is not as intense. In fact, some exercises in this category is pretty safe for people with potential health risks. Walking at a moderate pace every day is considered one of the safest forms of steady state cardio exercises.

There are definitely safety concerns with regard to HIIT training. Remember that unlike most exercises in steady state cardio, you will be pushing the pace really far away from your usual comfort zone. It's like taking your usual cardio and stepping it up about ten times faster (only a rough estimate).

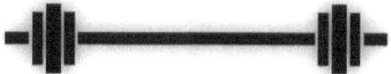

HIIT and Steady State Cardio Safety Concerns

As stated earlier, there are safety concerns when it comes to HIIT whereas there are very minimal safety concerns for most cardio. If you live a sedentary lifestyle and do very little exercise, then high intensive interval training will not exactly be a feasible first option. The same rule applies to people who have gone through periods of inactivity as well.

Get a Medical Clearance First

People who have a family history of heart disease, who are obese, diabetic or pre-diabetic, hypertension, and have a history of smoking should first seek to get a medical clearance from their doctors before they try any form of HIIT training.

That should be an appropriate safety measure for anyone with health risks or other medical conditions. When they call or describe something as "intense" then you should bet your bottom dollar that you will need a lot of preparation before you can engage in that sport or workout. Well, this rule actually applies to people with health risks no matter what form of exercise they will try to engage in.

Chances of Getting Injured

Now, this is the question that some people would like to ask. When you take an exercise, let's say running, and you run in full intensity – is there a higher risk of injury? The answer is in the affirmative; especially if you start running at full exertion and you haven't done any running for quite a while.

Of course, the idea is to do exercises with a graduated approach. That means you custom tailor the intensity to your fitness level. It is easier to lower the intensity of steady state cardio. For instance, if running is just too much of an exercise for you, you can just opt for a brisk-walk instead which is comparably easier on your body.

Heart Attack Risk

This is one of the big fears in some people's minds. Add to that the incident with sports news reporter Andy Marr who died of a stroke after doing rowing exercises. If you follow the news that went rambling at the time, it was suggested that too much strenuous exercise caused his death.

Add to that the prospects of doing "intense" exercise then you have here the perfect recipe for fear. It should be noted that it is possible to get a stroke doing any exercise – especially if it is prolonged or very intense.

If anything, the guys lifting a lot of weight in gyms should be at a higher risk. They're the ones who are doing the most intense workouts. In the case of Andy Marr, investigators found out that he was under a lot of stress and he also previously experienced a silent stroke.

The prolonged stress and strain from rowing took its toll on him and elevated his blood pressure. It was theorized that the blood vessels along his neck gave in due to the pressure, stress, and damage caused by the earlier stroke.

Nevertheless, we can never really know for sure. In theory, it is possible to experience a stroke whether doing HIIT or steady state cardio. Any exercise that elevates your heart rate and blood pressure is a candidate. That is why everyone should take the usual advice: seek the professional medical opinion before engaging in any kind of exercise.

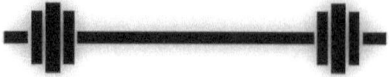

The Challenge of the Training Motivates

Some people get bored at doing the same exercise routine over and over again. Well, you may get bored at jogging 30 minutes every other day (some people do it every day). That is not the case with HIIT. The exercises are usually timed and your performance for each set is measured, which gives you a certain sense of competing with yourself – some people compete with each other when they do HIIT workouts in groups.

The challenge helps people stay motivated. And when a person's performance is measured and reported, their output usually increases (in some cases in exponential terms).

Cardiovascular Adaptations

Does the body's cardiovascular system adapt when one makes exercise a regular activity? The answer is yes. The adaptations include increased maximal oxygen consumption, also known as VO2max, increased cardiac contractility, increases in left ventricle heart mass, and improved stroke volume. These cardiovascular adaptations

Time Factor

With steady state exercises, you will have to do the same routine for a longer period of time. Some people don't have that time. In exchange for total amount of time spent, you can do the exercises in shorter time with HIIT.

Differences in Metabolic Adaptations

We have mentioned excess post exercise oxygen consumption or EPOC earlier. In a 2006 review by Laforgia and Gore, it was noted that HIIT produces more EPOC values compared to aerobic training (LaForgia, J., Withers, R.T., and Gore, C.J. (2006). Effects of exercise intensity and duration on the excess post-exercise oxygen consumption. Journal of Sports Science, 24(12), 1247-1264).

That means metabolic factors in body's cells remain hard at work after intense exercises have been performed. These muscle cells work hard to restore both metabolic and physiological conditions back to pre-exercise levels.

In effect after undergoing HIIT training, the body will increase in mitochondrial density – which is a type of metabolic adaptation. When that happens the body metabolizes fat as fuel instead of carbs. Remember that the mitochondria is the energy factory or powerhouse of the human cell. The higher the mitochondrial density, the higher the body's power or energy production – thus more ATP is produced and more body fat and carbs are burned.

One review shows that after 6 weeks of intense physical training, the participants of one study experienced higher fat burning compared to carbohydrate burning. Now, some studies suggest that the same results can be achieved in as few as two weeks only. Now, this increased fatty acid oxidation of course is achievable with high intensity interval training (Horowitz J.F. and Klein S. (2000). Lipid metabolism during endurance exercise. American Journal of Clinical Nutrition. 72(2 Suppl), 558S-563S).

Skeletal Muscle Adaptation

We have mentioned earlier that undergoing intense training (such as HIIT) can increase the body's mitochondrial density. That particular phenomenon actually has another benefit other than an increase in the body's ATP production (aka fat burning). You see, when the body's mitochondrial density increases you should expect the levels of mitochondrial enzymes increase as well, which helps to improve the body's skeletal muscle metabolic function. Of course, the same effect can be seen in steady state exercises but the enzyme levels are much higher after HIIT compared to other forms of cardio.

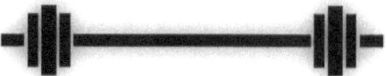

Which Type is Applicable to All Folks?

Now, here is another critical question. Although it can be said that anyone should be able to do HIIT, saying that only considers the most doable of scenarios. Almost anyone can do running intervals like running at full capacity then followed by a slow regular walk in the next phase. However, people with injury or are still aching will find HIIT a little too much.

That is why a lot of coaches only implement HIIT workouts about 2 to 3 days a week. On top of that, these workouts have their own training schedules apart from your regular training schedules. The level of difficulty of the workouts in HIIT can sometimes turn people off, which is why some people quit.

As we can see, HIIT has advantages over regular cardio and there are instances where regular steady state aerobic exercises are much more applicable. Although we emphasize the advantages of high intensity interval training in this book, it should also be pointed out that a well-rounded training is still the best option for anyone who is trying to lose weight and gain some serious muscle.

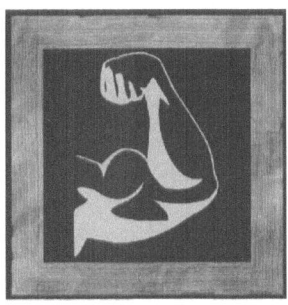

Chapter 3

HIIT Misconceptions

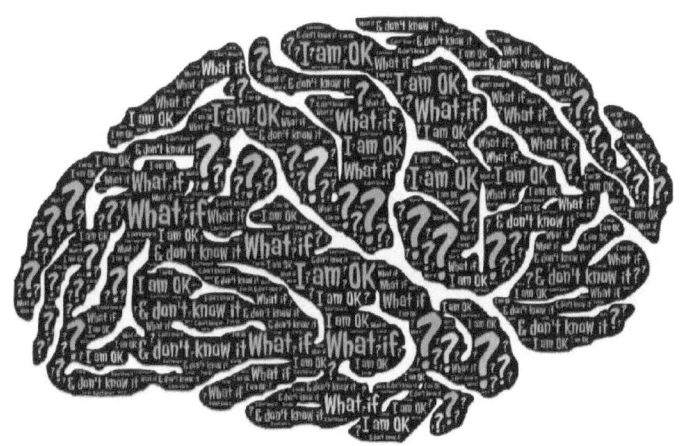

Now, before we move forward in the discussion of high intensity interval training, we should go over some of the most common misconceptions that people have about HIIT workouts. Yes, this type of interval training does have a lot of advantages but if you follow any of the myths mentioned below your performance may suffer. Well, sometimes you're just wasting time and effort needlessly.

HIIT Misconception #1 – Longer is Always Better

Some people believe that they can get more results from HIIT training by extending the periods of their workout by a few minutes or more – or even doubling the total workout time if possible. Maybe they think that the same principles in steady state cardio can apply in HIIT.

However, the fact of the matter is that you don't need those extra minutes. Well, you can even wonder if anyone can last more 60 minutes of straight high intensity exercises. Going at it for 30 minutes straight is already an enormous challenge even for the best athletes out there.

Here's a practical rule of thumb that you should remember: the longer you engage in a high intensity exercise, the faster the actual intensity of your exercise diminishes. That means if you extend your usual 15 minute HIIT routine to 30 minutes, you will no longer be efficiently exercising after you hit the 15 minute mark.

Your body will begin to tire. You will begin to feel the pain. In short, you will not be performing optimally. Let's face it. By the time you've hit the last minute of your HIIT workout for that day, your next repetition won't be as intense as it was when you started.

The effect of course is that the results you want to get gets diminished the longer you stay engaged in HIIT training. Be smart when it comes to your workout. That's the way to go.

If the routine is 20 minutes, then stick with the 20 minute routine. You will be getting more results that way than going beyond your natural ability or strength. Remember, don't work out more than you have strength.

HIIT Misconception #2 – All Kinds of Exercise is Suited for HIIT Training

Not all exercises are suitable for HIIT training. What you're looking for is an exercise that is really intense. Here's a test: if you are still able to talk while doing the said exercise then it's not intense enough. A truly intense work out or exercise is something that is so taxing that you need to focus on it. You will be hard pressed to breathe in the process.

That means exercises that focus on a single muscle won't cut it. Isolation exercises can't be used for HIIT. You can't do only bicep curls and hope to achieve a really intense workout. What you're supposed to be looking for are exercises that engage your body's full range of movement.

You need to choose exercises that build strength endurance that can also tax your body's cardiovascular system. Exercises that workout entire muscle groups should be in your list. Good examples of exercises that can be incorporated into HIIT training include hill sprints, sprint intervals, rower intervals, kettlebell presses, kettlebell cleans, dumbbell snatches, kettlebell swings, and burpees among other things. Remember – single joint exercises aren't for HIIT.

HIIT Misconception #3 –HIIT Training Alone Can Shed Fat

People have been shedding fat for quite a while using other forms of workouts before HIIT came along. People have been losing weight using steady state cardio for decades and there are folks who have been successful at it too. There are a lot of people who have been weight training and have shed lots of pounds – no miracle needed there either.

That should pretty much bust this myth altogether. However, there are two other parts to this misconception that we should also address. One part is that HIIT is all the training you need so you can lose body fat.

Well, that is true to a sense but you just can't discount the other exercises and training. Think of HIIT as one tool that will help you lose weight and build muscle. It's not your only tool and you can achieve your goals with the help of this tool but it's not the only tool that you will ever need to lose weight.

Okay, so what's the other part? If you do incorporate HIIT into your exercise regimen and sneak in a cheat meal after every workout session then don't expect to see a better figure next time you look in the mirror.

Remember that you can never outrun that biggie sized burger and fries with a sundae cone on the side. Don't assume that the EPOC effect that occurs after an HIIT exercise is a license to eat more. Poor eating habits won't give you the results you need. As a rule of thumb: 80% of your workout is done in the kitchen.

HIIT Misconception #4 –HIIT Training Will Bulk You Up Eventually

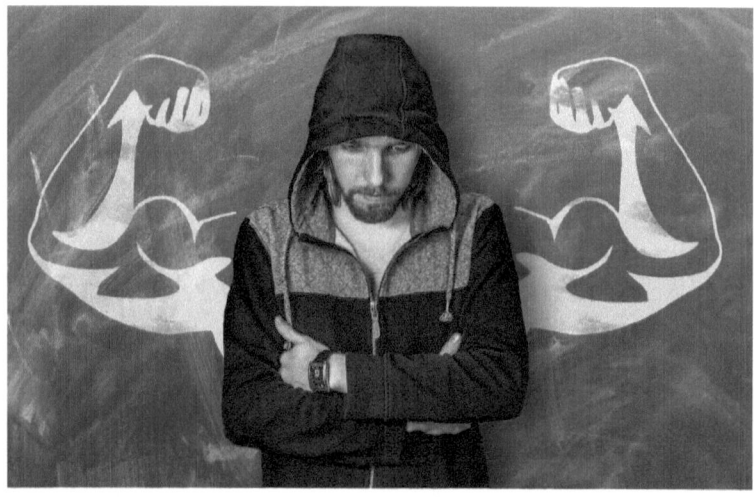

If you're looking to bulk up and buff up your figure into a new muscular you, then you're looking at the wrong workout. Remember that HIIT workouts aren't for building muscle mass like weight training does. It's not a substitute for that.

Again, here's what this type of training regimen is for: maintain and strengthen lean muscles, helps burn fat, improve your work capacity, improve your cardio, and increase your endurance. If you want to build some serious muscle then add some weight training to your workouts.

Remember that HIIT can improve your work capacity. That means it helps you work out at different intensities. Improved work capacity also allows you to do your workouts much longer. Bulking up requires something else – it's called muscular hypertrophy. That kind requires weights.

So don't be afraid to add some weighted compound exercises in your routine. A heavy dumbbell snatch set, kettlebell exercises, and other weight training will be quite helpful to you if you want to bulk up.

HIIT Misconception #5 – You Need Some Sort of Fancy Equipment

Did someone try to sell you something like some new exercise equipment so you can do HIIT workouts? Here's a hint: you don't need that to do HIIT training. You may want to incorporate some sort of weights later on. Your body will adjust to the intensity of your workouts and get stronger.

To keep challenging yourself, you may need to add weights like a kettlebell, ankleweights, or something. But you don't really need them to do HIIT as in essentially need them. Remember that the focus of this type of training is to increase your heart rate and keep it at that enhanced rate.

HIIT Misconception #6 – Anyone Can Do HIIT

Not everyone can run a marathon, that's a fact. Every marathon runner needs to prepare for that kind of a sporting event. It can even mean months of training which will prep your body for a feat of endurance of that magnitude.

You can say the same thing about HIIT training. If you haven't done any kind of exercise for a while then you may have to prepare yourself before undergoing an exercise routine that is labelled as "intense." You need to work on building your base fitness first.

That doesn't mean that doing HIIT is absolutely out of reach. It only means that you need to condition your body for it beforehand. In fact, you can even ease into it so to speak.

A session of HIIT will usually last 15 minutes up to half an hour on average. If you're just starting out, you won't be able to go all 30 minutes straight on full intensity. What you can do is to switch things up a little – well, it's not going to be a completely 100% HIIT training but your version will be the most challenging exercise given your fitness level.

At first you can do 5 minutes of intense workouts and then maybe 10 minutes of rest. You're going to need that much time to catch your breath. Remember, beginners can extend the rest times and then shorten the workout periods. The important thing is to allow your body to adapt to the intensity of the workout slowly.

Now, if you have any underlying medical conditions especially if it's really serious, you should first consult your doctor if HIIT is feasible for you. No one will blame you if you can't do HIIT.

HIIT Misconception #7 – HIIT is the Magic Exercise for Spot Reducing

Some people do kettlebell swings like there is no tomorrow. Well, the idea is to perform certain exercises that workout the core in the hopes of getting rid of the belly bulge. That's called spot reducing. Now, here's the deal: spot reducing just isn't possible.

Spot reducing is a myth. It doesn't matter what kind of exercise you're doing not even HIIT training is going to help you target that specific area you're aiming for. Even if you train a certain muscle group in the hopes of reducing the amount of fat on that area, HIIT will still not make a single difference.

All weight loss and fat burning plans should be designed as a form of total body fat loss strategy. You can't turn HIIT into a belly fat loss, or an arm flab fat loss, or some other kind of specific body part fat loss program. It just isn't going to work. Remember, aim for total fat loss – that beer gut will go away eventually.

HIIT Misconception #8 – HIIT is Only for the Fat Loss Phase

It is absolutely up to you if you really want to have some sort of cardio when you're in the muscle building phase. However, you should know that it isn't a must. It's actually all up to you. Your HIIT training should have a separate schedule and it should be in conjunction with your workout schedule.

There are benefits to sticking with your HIIT training schedule even if it falls in the other phases of your training. Forgoing HIIT training simply because you're on the muscle gain phase will create some fat gains – remember, you're already consuming a calorie surplus.

Remember that HIIT is a pretty darn good workout and it burns a lot of body fat. Simply put, it will help prevent any fat gains. It will help offset some of the extra fat that you will have otherwise gained in the process.

HIIT Misconception #9 – It's Just Some form of Cardio

Some people dismiss HIIT training as just some form of cardio. As we have pointed out so far, it's actually more than that. On the other hand, some people just do cardio exercises for their HIIT training. Remember that you can also do strength training as well as sports centric exercises for your HIIT workout. If done correctly, your endurance will increase and you will eventually feel stronger and then burn fat along the way.

HIIT Misconception #10 – It Should Replace All Cardio Workouts

Saying that everyone should abandon regular cardio and just focus on HIIT is pushing everything to the extreme. Now here's something that you should know – if you abandon regular cardio in lieu of an HIIT only training you will lose cardiovascular endurance.

Sure you can go ballistic for a minute or two, but you won't last. You're not going to have the endurance to run for a full 60 minutes if the only exercises you do are HIIT exercises.

Regular cardio is great for warm ups and cool downs. They should also be the exercise of choice during your recovery days. Slow cycling and jogging will help you burn some calories whilst giving your body a time to rest and recover.

My Favorite HIIT Misconception – You're Too Old to do HIIT

This is my favorite misconception about HIIT training. People who have tried HIIT once or twice may complain about how difficult it is and will at times think that this kind of training will kill their grandparents.

First off, if you do HIIT correctly, you're not going to kill yourself. If you're old and you haven't done any exercises in a while then you should start with an exercise routine that will be easier for you. But, as stated earlier, you can water things down a bit in preparation for true blue HIIT. You can prepare yourself slowly, building up your strength, and then eventually do some HIIT training. It applies to everyone from ages 16 to 60, so to speak (pun intended).

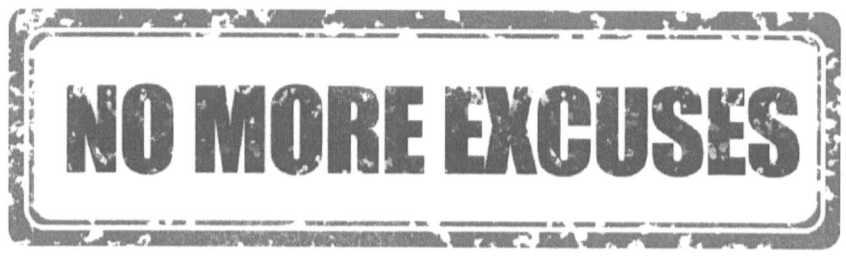

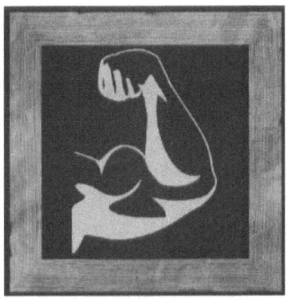

Chapter 4

How Often Should You Train

HIIT workouts will give you some serious revved up metabolism when done correctly. However, in order to reap the benefits from this training method, you should know how to execute it properly and you should also adhere to your schedule. A common question asked is how often should one train in HIIT? We'll cover that in this chapter.

Your Fitness Goal and Your Fitness Level

You need to consider both your fitness level and your fitness goals when you figure out how much HIIT training you should incorporate into your current training routine. Remember that you will be doing one of the hardest training methods ever conceived.

It actually combines two types of fat burning workouts. The first one is high intensity training. The second one is interval training. Both types of training are already pretty tough on their own – but now you're combining the two.

Working at Newbie and Couch Potato Levels

If you are the type of person who has just decided to part ways with his beloved couch (with chips on the side of course) then you should take it easy. HIIT includes interval training, which can take a toll on your heart.

And because you will be doing a lot of high intensity exercises, you will first need to condition your body. Introduce workouts gradually. These workouts should be carefully scheduled – a fitness trainer should or your doctor should help you determine what exercises you are ready for.

Doing bursts of intense cardio will be too hard for beginners and anyone who has done zero workouts for many years. You should be doing low intensity workouts first like walking on a treadmill, jogging, or use an elliptical trainer. You should do that and become comfortable with it before you explore the possibilities of HIIT.

Moderately Active Lifestyles

If you live a moderately active lifestyle – that means you are working out on certain days or you engage in some form of physical activity on a regular basis, then you can add HIIT training to your schedule up to two to three times a week. By moderately active we are talking about someone who is physically active anywhere from two to four times a week. You can even add low intensity cardio in your routine, if your goal is to improve your heart health.

If your goal is weight loss, then add either strength training or some metabolic resistance workouts to your HIIT training workouts. Experts suggest that strength training added to HIIT workouts make for one of the most optimal methods for anyone who wants to lose weight.

People with Active Lifestyles

Those who are already living active lifestyles will enjoy the challenge brought by HIIT training. If you are serious about getting a better figure and a healthier circulatory system then this type of training should be a welcome challenge to you.

The bursts in interval training and frequency of the workouts will be enough to spice up an already boring training routine. To make things even more interesting, you can vary the work-rest ratios while you're at it.

For active folks, doing HIIT two to three days a week should be enough to fill in the gaps. If your goal is weight loss then you can add two to three sessions of strength training. If you feel that all of the HIIT isn't challenging enough then simply reduce the rest periods in between the bursts.

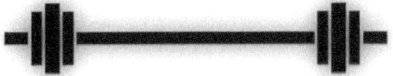

Some Reminders

Again, we should emphasize that the quality of your training is more important that the length of your training. You don't need to train longer when you're doing HIIT. Keep your HIIT workouts short and sweet. That will prevent the overtraining of your muscles.

Now, here's something that will cook your noodle. If you ask one expert he will tell you one training frequency and another expert will tell you another. Some will say it is okay to do some HIIT three times a week no matter what your fitness level is.

Some will tell you that you should train four times a week if you really want to increase your body's oxygen uptake. However, there will be fitness experts who will tell you that you should match 1 day of HIIT with a day of steady state cardio and that should be performed once or twice a week.

Of course, that is simply the opinion of these fitness trainers. Here's a tip to help you make up your mind: be aware of your own personal comfort levels. For instance, if you have an HIIT session scheduled today and you're still aching from the workouts you did the day before then you should rather schedule a rest day.

You should give your body some time to adapt to the intensity of your training. Remember that it all depends on your fitness level and your fitness goals. HIIT will be as tough as a bitch the first time you try it.

It will hurt and you will feel sore and some people quit after trying it for the first time. But don't quit. Give it time. Enjoy your rest day and recover well. After you have recovered, hit it!

So, what happens after your body has adapted to the intensity of your interval training? One day your body will be able to take the punishment from HIIT. When that happens you should increase the frequency and/or intensity of your workouts by 10 percent. Increase the level of the challenge when your body has adapted to the current difficulty level.

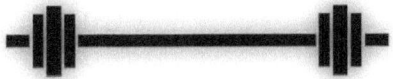

In Summary

Here's a little summary of what we have covered in this chapter. Note that the information below is a bare minimum and it is only suggested. The best way to go is to talk to your doctor or fitness trainer first. Discuss whether the schedules below will suit you or not:

Newbie/Couch Potato Fitness Level
(Those doing 0 to 2 workout days each week)

Goal: Better Heart Health	Do HIIT one day a week + cardio (low intensity)
Goal: Weight Loss	Do HIIT training one day each week + some low intensity cardio exercise
Goal: Maintain Muscle Mass	Not feasible

Semi Active Fitness Level
(Those doing 2 to 4 workout days a week)

Goal: Better Heart Health	Schedule HIIT sessions 1 or 2 days a week + 1 day of cardio (low intensity)
Goal: Weight Loss	Schedule HIIT sessions 2 to 3 days a week. + 1 day circuit training
Goal: Maintain Muscle Mass	Schedule HIIT sessions 2 days each week + schedule strength training 2 days each week.

Active Fitness Level
(Those doing 4 to 7 workout days each week)

Goal: Better Heart Health	Schedule HIIT sessions 2 days each week + 2 days of cardio (low intensity)
Goal: Weight Loss	Schedule HIIT sessions 2 to 3 days each week + 2 to 3 days of circuit training
Goal: Maintain Muscle Mass	Schedule HIIT sessions 2 days each week + schedule strength

	training 3 to 4 days each week

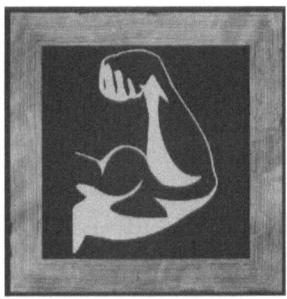

Chapter 5

How to Incorporate HIIT Into Your Workout

You can't just jump into a high intensity interval training regimen even if you are already doing some cardio. In the previous chapter we talked about scheduling your HIIT workouts and how much you should be doing based on several factors.

It should be emphasized here that HIIT workouts are so intense that you can risk injuring yourself if you do things carelessly. So, be careful. Now, even though your risk for injury is pretty low, you're still at risk for overtraining and burnout if you're not careful.

We'll go over how to incorporate HIIT workouts safely into your current training. The tips and information below will help even if you are just starting out. The important thing is that you plan things well and stick to your routine. Of course, there will be exceptions and we'll go over those as well.

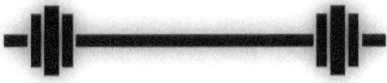

Easing Into It

Approaching things from the point of view of someone who hasn't done any kind of workout or exercise, how should you begin? The first step of course is to gain a baseline fitness level. When we say baseline fitness level, we're referring to your aerobic fitness. That of course includes better heart health and better respiratory health.

If you haven't done any exercises then you should begin by working on your aerobic fitness. You should first commit to 20 minutes of cardio. Schedule that three times a week (i.e. you'll be working out 3 days in a week and spending 20 minutes exercising on your workout days).

To establish your aerobic fitness level, you should be religiously doing your cardio workouts for about a month. That should be enough to help you get your minimum cardio fitness. After a month's work on steady state cardio like jogging, cycling, walking, or any other kind of regular cardio you should introduce intervals into your routine – that way your workout days won't be so boring you will quit. Overtime, you can increase the intensity of your workouts as well.

At the start, you won't be doing the full blown version of an HIIT session. So, how do you add the intervals into your usual steady state cardio? Here's how. Do your steady state cardio – you pick the type of exercise you like of course. Now, add two or three intervals after a month of doing that. Just 30 seconds per interval into the mix.

Now, that will make your training a bit more difficult than usual. It may take some time before you become fully comfortable with intervals included in your workout, but you'll get there. Eventually after a few weeks of that your body's physical conditioning will improve and you can do intervals without any issues.

Once you're at that point, you can add more intervals into your training sessions. After your warm up you can start with regular cardio and then insert 30 seconds of interval training in between. Keep doing that all throughout your training day. Of course, there should be no intervals during warm ups and cool downs.

When considering the intensity of your workouts, you should do your intervals at lower intensity. Just remember to spread out your interval training over the course of your entire workout session. Remember to keep the times short and the intensity low – at this stage you're not ready for the real deal just yet. Don't push your luck.

Now, spreading out your intervals in between does not necessarily constitute a full blown HIIT session. What you're doing for now is increasing your body's stamina. You'll need that later when you begin doing 100% true blue brutal HIIT.

In the following month after you have established your base aerobic fitness level you should allow your body to adapt to this kind of training. Listen to your body. Heed what it is telling you. Also, pay attention to how long you recover. Some people recover quickly while others take an extra day or two. If you're still tired, in pain, or in slow motion mode, then take a day off the gym (or workout session if you have one scheduled).

Remember, all you're doing is easing yourself into it. The goal is to build your stamina at this point. Practice changing the speeds and rates of your cardio exercises. That will also help you prepare for the intense workouts you will be doing later. Slowly increase the intensity and slowly go for slightly longer intervals.

Keep Things Interesting

Some people start their way back into cardio exercises by walking or running. That of course depends on their fitness level and their personal interests. However, after doing the same kind of exercise for a month or so, some folks will get bored. There are people who quit working out simply because they get bored.

Keep things interesting. If you have come to a point where you are totally bored (or have come to hate) running then stop. Do something else. If you don't like a particular kind of exercise anymore, chances are it won't become a habit. You should find a workout that you enjoy. We have already mentioned several exercises that will work well with HIIT in a previous chapter. You can choose any of those if you like.

Of course, you can also look around for some new exercise that you might want to try. You can even cycle from one exercise to another if you like. Now, when you choose an exercise or workout you should pick the ones that work the larger muscle groups. An example of which are your legs. Exercises and workouts of this kind can get your heart rate up fast. You should also choose the exercises that allow you to accelerate to top speed rather quickly and you should also decelerate the rate of the said exercise just as fast.

You can select exercises that are considered non-traditional. For instance, you can do as many burpees as you can for about 30 to 60 seconds. After doing that you can walk for 60 seconds or more. After you have rested, you can go back to burpees again.

The important thing is that you can do the exercises as fast as you can. You can mix any kind of interval exercise just to make things really interesting. The limit is your creativity.

The Smart Schedule

We have already mentioned that HIIT workouts have their own schedule. Some days of the week you will be engaged in your other workouts be it weight training, cardio, or some other kind of training you can think of. On other days you should be doing HIIT workouts.

Now, there is a certain issue that comes up every now and then. You see, it's pretty easy to overwork your legs when you switch from HIIT workout days to non-HIIT days. Sometimes you work your legs on an HIIT training day and forget that you're supposed to do weighted leg exercises in the gym the following day (also happens the other way around).

So, what happens? You walk into the gym with legs aching like no other. What had just happened? You over trained a body part that you were working on. That of course will impede your progress and will force you to call it in and take a rest and recovery day. It will hamper your recuperation efforts and a day like that will diminish whatever progress you have made so far.

Remember, plan your workouts well. You may want to keep your scheduled leg workouts at the gym as far away as possible from the scheduled HIIT training days. Allow at least 24 hours in between – that should be enough recovery for your legs. That of course will depend on how sore you are. If you're still sore then take a break – no one will blame you.

Note that HIIT can quickly deplete the glycogen levels in your muscles. Glycogen is the stored form of carbs (they're stored in your muscular tissues and these things power your workouts). Your leg day should be paired with low intensity steady state cardio day, which is the smart way to go.

And here's an exception that you should take note of – what if you're already a hard core gym guy, a bodybuilder in pre-contest condition? To answer that question, here's what you can do: after a leg day at the gym, do some HIIT workouts. That will help your body tap into those deep seated fat stores.

Now here's a caveat: you should only do that if you're an advanced athlete. If you're preparing for competition, then that may be a pretty good idea. But if you're new or on the intermediate level, you may be just kidding yourself; you don't want to face that kind of punishment.

VINCENT BLACKSHEAR

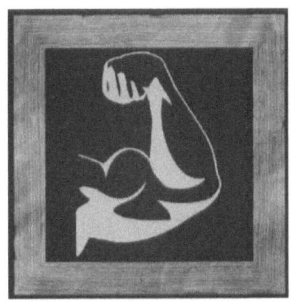

Chapter 6

Making the Most of Your Training

In this chapter we'll look at some of the tips that may be of use to you in case you want to incorporate high intensity interval training in your overall workout. Pay attention to the reminders mentioned below. They may help make things easier for you.

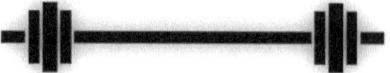

Don't Forget to Fuel Up

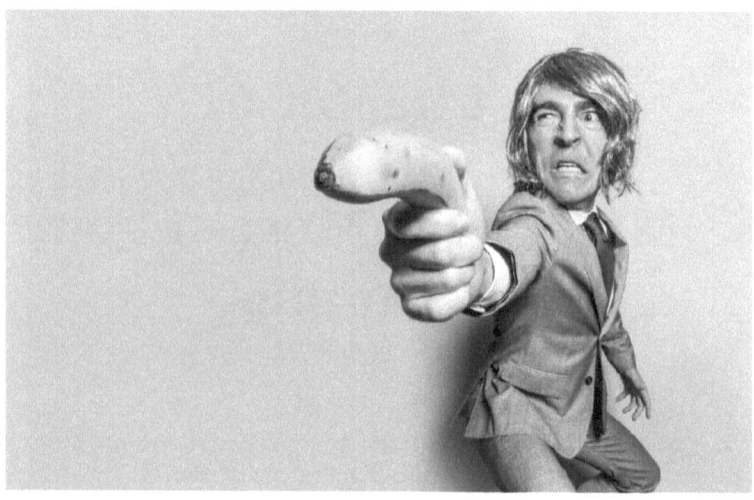

Some people forget to fuel up before they begin an HIIT workout. There are those who neglect this part of working out. That is definitely a big mistake. Remember that HIIT is a really intense way torch fat from your body. It's not some run off the mill exercise (pun intended there).

Even professional athletes take the time to prepare well for this kind of workout – that includes eating right. If those buff and superb athletic types feel the burn and get tired due to HIIT, then you should prepare well yourself.

According to the American Council on Exercise, you should be eating something from a moderately high card meal to an actual high carb meal before engaging in an HIIT session. According to them, you should be eating this carb rich meal 30 minutes before the actual workout.

Pre-Workout Munch

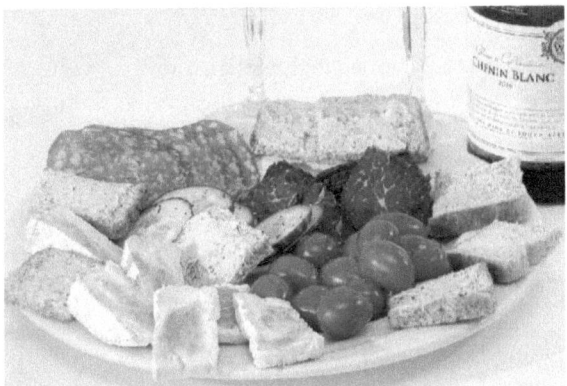

Due to the intensity of HIIT workouts, it is vital that you follow a healthy and nutritious diet. Since you are working out, you should be on a moderate level to a high level carbohydrate rich diet. Of course, since you're trying to build some muscle along the way, then you should include a good amount of protein.

Here are a few suggestions that you can try:
1. Almonds and other dried fruits
2. Cottage cheese, Greek yogurt (non-fat), and other fruits
3. Toast (use whole wheat bread) + peanut butter + banana or any other fruit

Post Workout Munch

Don't be afraid to eat something after you're done working out. Remember that you need to replace the glycogen or energy stores in your muscle tissue. The food you eat post workout will also be used by your body for muscle repair.

After undergoing HIIT training, the muscles you have just worked out will need a lot of rest and repair. Studies show that a combination of protein and carbohydrates after some serious workout will help replenish depleted energy stores and help the body begin repairing muscle fibers.

You should have something to eat within 30 minutes after undergoing a

HIIT session. Research also tells us that the ratio of carbs to proteins at this point should be at 3:1. This boosts the glycogen production and it helps prepare the body for the next workout you may be doing.

So, what can you eat post HIIT workout? Here are a few suggestions:
1. Any of the suggested food mentioned in the pre-workout section earlier.
2. Pita bread dipped in hummus.
3. Cheese, fruit, and whole wheat crackers.
4. Soy milk, fruit, and whole grain cereal.

Remember that you need to approach HIIT workout sessions as if they are weight training sessions. You won't have enough energy to lift a lot of weights if you didn't fuel up before you walk into the gym, right? You will need a meal in you first! As a rule, pre-workout nutrition is your gateway to obtaining optimal performance when you do HIIT workouts. Well, that rule also applies for weightlifting, strength and conditioning, or any other intense workout you may have scheduled.

Now, here's another thing that you should remember. The closer you are to your actual training time the more you should stick to easily digestible carbs and proteins. You want food that your body can digest quickly. But if you have some time like a few hours or so, you can opt for whole foods.

As stated earlier, the food you eat in your pre-workout meals will be the fuel for your muscles and it will also supply the amino acids for rebuilding broken down muscle fibers.

There will be times when you won't really need a lot of carbs to get through your workout – that is even if you are going to lift some weights. That may also apply to days when the goal is to torch some fat. Going for about 10 to 20 grams of carbs for such days may already be enough to fuel you through an entire workout session including HIIT.

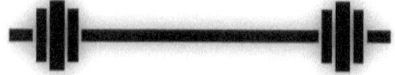

Let Your Body Take the Lead

We can't emphasize this point enough – you should listen to what your body is telling you. Don't force it, work with your body. If the fatigue is still so intense the day when you're supposed to do HIIT or do some other workout at the gym then switch up your schedule. Use that day as a rest day instead.

If you want you can also just go for some steady state cardio at low intensity. That way you don't have to mess up your schedule that much. At least you got something done. However, you should watch out and don't overdo it. You don't want to over train especially when you are already sore.

You will be more efficient during your training session if you are properly rested. In short, you will get more done that way than merely just forcing yourself. Again, the quality of your workout is more important than the length or amount of training you have done.

Beginners will usually do only one HIIT session each week. That means they can do some other form of exercise in the days ahead before their scheduled HIIT training day. To help them prepare for their scheduled HIIT training day, they can do some intervals in lower intensities.

Another way to help prepare you for the rigors of intense intervals is to do resistance training. Your body will adapt to that level of stress and help you become more efficient when you engage in intense intervals. You can then add more intense and longer intervals in your preparation stage.

Now, during your non-HIIT days, you should still pay attention to your recovery. Give your body enough time to recover. If you're a beginner you don't want to push it too far. There should be at least 24 hours of rest in between a non-HIIT day and the actual HIIT training day.

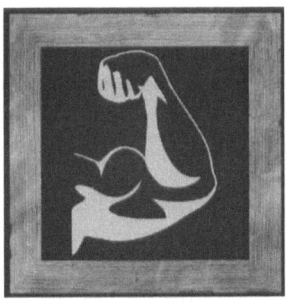

Chapter 7

To HIIT or not to HIIT, This is Not Blackjack

Training, any sort of training, will eventually result in pain. Well, you are tearing through muscle fibers which will hurt later on by the way. On top of that, you will feel your body make huge demands for oxygen. You'll be gasping for air when you do HIIT training. It ranks as one of the most difficult training methods anywhere.

HIIT will demand a lot from you and sometimes right in the middle of it all you will just want to stop. Some may even ask if the pain is worth it? Of course we all know the answer to that question but you have to answer that question yourself. It's as subjective a question as it can be.

Now, there are times when HIIT training isn't the best idea for your training day. There are certain situations when you really have to skip HIIT workouts and it will be the better decision for you. We'll go over that in this section of this book.

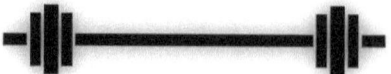

Have You Considered Your Diet?

One of the first things that you should look into is your diet. Yes, your diet will dictate whether you should be engaging in HIIT workouts or not. What type of diet plan are you on? There are diets that have low to zero carbs on it. If you're on that kind of diet then the smart move is not to undergo a HIIT session.

Attempting to do a HIIT workout without seeing even a slice of bread or any kind of carb for several weeks is a bad idea. You will be setting yourself up for a loss of lean muscle mass and that is nothing short of a disaster. On top of that, your muscles will not have enough glycogen to even complete your workout.

Sure there are other sources of energy that your body can use such as different types of protein, but your body's main source of energy comes from carbs. Your body will naturally tap into that resource when your metabolic systems are stressed. It will tap into whatever source of energy it can find. You may find out the hard way that you can't complete your HIIT session without having some sort of carbs on your diet.

Now, if you have a reduced carb diet, you may still run into problems. Your calorie levels maybe too low and you will still have difficulty completing your workout. Note that in the effort to get rid of fat, your body will still need some sort of fuel to get the workouts done. You need glucose and you will need carbs. No carbs, no HIIT session. It's that simple.

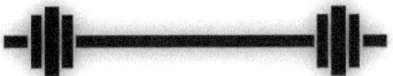

Intensity and Weight Workout Volume

What does your weight workout look like? This is another thing that you should look into when you're considering whether you are supposed to do a HIIT session or not. Are there times when you feel that your strength is just lagging and everything is in slow motion mode? Did you check your workout volume in your previous weight lifting day?

Let's say you just did legs the day before – yeah you feel pumped up and you think you can do some heavy lifting with your upper body. You decide to do some hard back workouts – not a bad combination, right? But why is it that you're having difficulty doing back exercises?

Here's why. Your central nervous system has broken down. Some people make this huge error in judgment when scheduling their workout days. They will do high volume lifting workouts one day – that is already a highly intensive work out by the way.

On top that they will also do two sessions of HIIT training; that's on their off-gym day. Sometimes they will even add an upper body workout and time a HIIT session a few hours later. That doesn't sound so bad doesn't it?

You're mixing things up and you're working different parts of your body so one workout shouldn't interfere with the other, right? Have you considered the intensity of the workouts? What about the workout volume? Doing high intense training will tax your CNS – your central nervous system.

Remember that just like the rest of your body's metabolic systems, your CNS can only take so much. It has a limit too. If you give it too much to handle then you will end up struggling in your next workout session. And that's why after doing one intense workout session after another, you feel like everything is in slow motion.

Change the intensities of your workouts. That's the way to go. If you have to go through a rest day then do it. Give your body's systems some time to recover. Remember that it's not your back muscles that are fatigued – your CNS is. Your CNS determines your actual strength output.

Now, when you're doing a HIIT session, you will be giving your CNS ten times the stress of a regular cardio session. That means you can't do HIIT sessions when you're already doing a lot of high volume weight training. Your CNS will get taxed out and then it will tap out. You're just not going to be as efficient as you want to be. That's why you experience the symptoms of an overtraining syndrome.

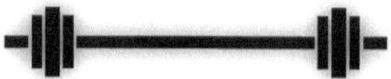

Your Ability to Recover

Different people have different recovery rates. It is critical that you observe your body's ability to recover. Now this is the bad news – if you observe that your body has a really poor recovery system then HIIT workouts may not really be a good option for you at all. If that is the case then talk to your doctor and your fitness coach. See if you can explore other options.

Now, what if your recovery system is good? If that is the case consider adding HIIT sessions gradually. Never push yourself beyond what you can naturally do. Some people push themselves too much to the point of overtraining. They give up on HIIT training eventually and will say that it's not for them. Let's emphasize this point we've made in a previous chapter – ease yourself into it.

These are the factors that you should consider when you're trying to decide whether to HIIT or not to HIIT. It's not the easiest training method out there and you don't want to burn yourself out because of that. However, you may be missing out on the benefits of HIIT sessions if you make the wrong decisions about your training. If it's time to skip a session then skip – it's all for your own good.

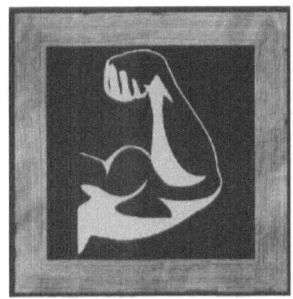

Conclusion

Thank you for downloading this book. I hope this book was able to convince you that HIIT is a great way to maximize the benefits of your current workout sessions. The next step is to evaluate how you can safely incorporate HIIT training into your current exercise regimen.

To get you started in incorporating HIIT into your regimen, try going into Youtube for some beginner level exercises. The channel "The Body Coach TV" is a good channel to ease your way into HIIT and not get overwhelmed. You can also try using the Youtube search bar and type in "HIIT for beginners".

The Youtube channel and videos are not mine and I have no connection to the owner. It is just a recommendation, and you are always free to find your own.

VINCENT BLACKSHEAR

ABOUT THE AUTHOR

Vincent Blackshear

Vincent Blackshear is a nurse, a volunteer firefighter and paramedic. He was born in a family that fostered his preference for physical activities, which led him to his first love — sports.

He's a father, an athlete since grade school, and a passionate health buff. He believes that changing the world and making a difference starts with oneself. Having that mind set, he strongly advocates exercise and keeping oneself healthy. The primary step to health is creating good eating habit and a regular exercise routine. He wants to share the benefits of exercise and get people to be in their top form, so that they too can make a difference. Let's change the world one step at a time!